Dental Coaching Provided by Coach Ike Rahimi, DMD

Coach Ike offers seminars for dental professionals and their teams. Search Amazon.com for more books from Coach Ike, and discover how he can help you!

Coach Ike Rahimi, DMD
- Doctor Leadership
- Dental Staff Training
- Practice Management
- Profit Building
- Modern Communications

Copyright ©2017 Ike Rahimi, DMD
All Rights Reserved. This publication and any content herein may not be reproduced in any way, shape, form or format, digitally or otherwise, without the express written permission of Ike Rahimi.

Table of Contents

Preface — 5

1. Set Up For Success — 9
- I. Mission Statement and Vision — 9
- II. Marketing — 10
- III. Company Culture — 12
- IV. Great Companies, Great Cultures — 16
- V. Millennials in the Workforce — 17

2. Mastering Leadership Skills — 19
- I. Be Fluid — 20
- II. Be Open-Minded — 20
- III. Invest Time in People — 21
- IV. Focus on What's Important — 21
- V. Have a Game Plan — 22
- VI. Be Aware — 22
- VII. Know When to Say "No" — 23

3. Defining Job Positions — 25
- I. Staff Roles — 25
- II. Punctuality and Social Media — 27
- III. Employee Requirements — 27

4. Crafting the Optimal Help-Wanted Ad — 35
- I. The Impactful Ad — 35
- II. What to Include — 36
- III. Sample Ad — 37
- IV. Targeting the Candidates — 38
- V. Employment Ad Venues — 39

5. Before the Interview — 41
- I. Don't Rush! — 41
- II. Previewing and Resumes — 42
- III. The Five Steps to Review a Resume — 43

6. Conducting the Interview — 47
- I. Behavioral Interviews — 47
- II. Leadership and Mediation — 48
- III. Team Players and Problem Solvers — 49
- IV. The Four Types of Dental Interviews — 50
- V. The Final Review — 54

7. Introducing the Newest Team Member — 55
- I. Encourage Acceptance — 55
- II. The New Employee's Life Story — 56
- III. Employee Manual — 56
- IV. Your Employees are Your Best Trainers — 57
- V. In the Beginning, Be a Guide — 58
- VI. Patient Care Matters to Every Employee — 59
- VII. Don't Forget About the Fun Stuff — 59
- VIII. Make Sure They Know: Change is Constant — 60

8. Training and Education — 61

9. A Full Employee Checklist — 63

10. Ten Questions Every Dental Office Must Answer — 69

Conclusion — 91

Preface

Once finished with dental school, I was eager to go out and make things happen. I had lived on a meager student budget for years and was excited to finally make some money and buy cool things. I envisioned a well-run, remarkably productive dental office and assumed the practice would run fine by itself while also being a happy place to work.

At first I worked in practices owned by other dentists, and they had their own set ways of running their offices. After spending some time working for them, I was able to purchase my own practice. I bought an established practice with staff and patients already included. Sounds great, right?

I was young and full of energy and wanted to make significant improvements to the practice, yet the existing staff were set in their ways. For example, the first time I opened a Friday schedule, most of the staff objected. I gave in because I had no idea how to overcome conflict. In addition, I faced other team problems—not listening, not accepting new protocols, and playing political and power games.

For years I took a passive approach to leadership, assuming the practice was running fine as long as the bills were being paid. I didn't know how to improve the front area dynamics, how to build a good rapport with patients, or how to manage larger case files like for a full-mouth reconstruction. I was careful to avoid conflict because without the original staff I wouldn't be able to run my office.

I was the owner, yet I felt like an employee. I would come in, see patients, and leave. There were no leadership guidelines, no tips for group meetings, no ideas to inspire my team. Deep down, I wasn't content, because I knew that our practice could do so much better—so I started changing things. Unfortunately, while doing this I became more authoritarian, demanding that things get done. I started doing more enjoyable procedures and saw my revenues improve, however, my directive managerial style began causing negative feelings to develop among my employees.

I didn't realize that 80% of a dental office is run by the team. I didn't realize that the higher the level of rapport between my staff and my patients, the higher the case acceptance level would be. Other things that I learned: The longer employees had been in the dental field, the harder it was to change their bad habits, but more mature employees knew how to better communicate with patients. Conversely, younger team members often knew more about the technology, but lacked the people skills essential for building a successful practice.

The current state of dental practice is shifting. A recent report by the ADA stated that in the last 10 years, large corporate dental offices saw the biggest profits and growth while small private dental offices saw the least. I believe that over the next decade this gap will widen, and that 80% of patients will go to large dental offices because they take all forms of insurance and do a hard sell. The remaining 20% will go to private dental offices that deliver customized, stellar patient services. Dental care will continue to parallel the retail and service markets of other large and small businesses.

To provide customized, stellar service to *your* patients, you will need an effective, competent, and committed team. You may be the best clinician in the world but, without a great team to back you up, you can only do so much.

I hope to shed some light on developing a great team, starting from before the hiring process to the hiring process itself, and then talking about training and education.

- Coach Ike Rahimi, DMD

team [tem] (n.) - people gathered together and working in unison to achieve a common goal

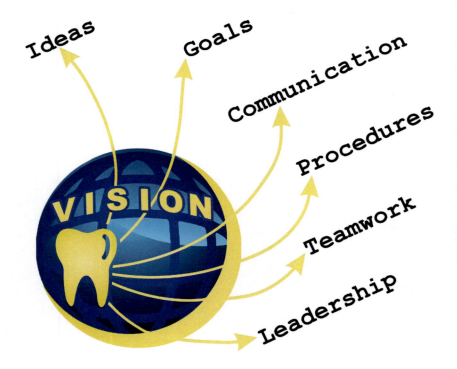

1   Set Up For Success

> *Be a yardstick of quality. Some people aren't used to an environment where excellence is expected.*
> — Steve Jobs

I. Mission Statement and Vision

Before anything can happen, your office must have a mission statement and a vision:

A mission statement describes what a company does now; a vision outlines what a company wants to be in the future. As the dental practice owner, you should develop the mission statement and the vision, perhaps in collaboration with key staff members.

Your mission statement should be clear and concise, and communicate the purpose and values of your office. A few sample mission statements are: "We proudly serve the public by licensing drivers, registering vehicles, securing identities, and regulating the motor vehicle industry." (the California Department of Motor Vehicles); "To build healthier lives, free of cardiovascular diseases and stroke." (the American Heart Association); and, "To inspire Americans to protect wildlife for our children's future." (the National Wildlife Federation).

Your vision should be an achievable, realistic aspiration. A few sample visions are: "To create a better every day life for the many people." (IKEA); "To become the nation's leading utility in the eyes of our customers, employees and shareholders." (Pacific Gas and Electric); "A trusted leader in delivering innovative DMV services." (the California Department of Motor Vehicles).

Please take this step seriously and don't just copy something off the Internet. What do you as a professional and your office as a dental care provider really stand for?

Once you have articulated a clear and meaningful mission statement and vision, your next step is to go about attracting patients.

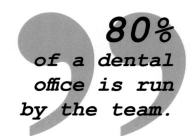

80% of a dental office is run by the team.

II. Marketing

You can market through Internet marketing companies, social media, direct mailers and print media, TV, radio, local theaters, and more. The benefit of this is that you will be able to present exactly the kind of image of yourself and your office that you want. The downsides are that advertising can get very pricey and the return on investment can often be very low.

Patient referral is asking your existing patients to refer others to your dental office. The benefit of this is that the costs are low and, when patients are referred this way, they are more likely to accept treatment plans.

As the leader of your dental office, you have to determine what message you want to send the public about your dental office. Are you advertising veneers, wisdom teeth extractions, or dental implants? Whatever you're advertising, the message has to be clear and your team has to understand and be on board with that message. What you want to do first is look at your return on investment. What procedures bring in the highest profits and have the highest patient satisfaction? Don't forget to include those procedures you really enjoy doing.

Here are my top five procedures:
- Traditional braces
- Dental implant placement and restorations
- Fillings
- Root canals
- Deep cleanings

Now that you have picked your favorite procedures, you need to have an advertising piece that is captivating, with great images and great catchphrases. You also need to have an advertising hook to give patients a reason to call. Whether you like it or not, offering a discount reduces barriers and increases the chances that potential patients will call.

With social media, review sites, and a plethora of digital gossip highways, we are constantly under scrutiny. On the one hand, such scrutiny makes our job more difficult but, on the other hand, we can benefit from developing a human-centric culture (employees, staff, and patients). By matching our team's skills with patient needs we can create an atmosphere of appreciation and reward.

Encourage your team to become more cognizant of the patient as a whole person, so that team members can act in a predictable and reliable way. For example, if your business is primarily working with low-income patients who rely on insurance, make sure that your team is sensitive to the sacrifices the patients have to make to see you. Likewise, if your office is doing a lot of braces, this attracts kids and teenagers, and your office should then be kid-friendly. And, if you focus on dentures, it would be prudent to have AARP magazines available in the waiting room and at least one staff member who is familiar with wearing some type of dentures.

It is important that your team be aware of what your goals are so that they can help work towards reaching them. When you win, your office wins, and your team wins. I have a system of rewards for certain goal levels and have set it in such a way that my staff hits the goal at least 75% of the time. In previous years my staff have won cash prizes, trips, and vacations. The most important part is that when you win, they win. You have to share some of your winnings with your team.

> *Everyone will work to keep your office thriving if they feel they are an integral part of it.*

III. Company Culture

Company culture is the personality of a company. It defines the environment in which employees work.

The best cultures make all employees feel safe and welcome. As business owners and health service providers both laws and human ethics bind us. Think about it for a minute:

how would you want to be treated if you were working for someone else? Would you like to be respected for your accomplishments? How should you be compensated? Is employer loyalty important to you? Do you feel good working in an office full of smiling patients and happy staff?

Have a system to reward employees for great work. I'm not talking about money but a simple "Thank you for your great effort today" or "Go team! You guys killed it today." How about fun team-building games for the team?

Outlining expectations and allowing employees to plan their own personal and professional growth gives them something to look forward to when they come to work. Dead-end jobs reduce personal incentives to develop. This leads to low employee morale, slack behavior, and apathy. Empowered employees strive for better performance and this in turn brings the entire team up.

By discussing mission statements and visions and protocols for the entire office, we can give the team tools for accountability.

The benefits of having a strong company culture are:

1. Team retention

> Your team is the most important variable in running an efficient and profitable dental office. Each team member has a different need; money isn't always the main driving force. It's important to include a system of benefits that is not solely monetary. In our office, if a staff member needs to bring his or her child to work in the case of an emergency, we have a room for childcare. If someone is ill, we ask that they stay home and get better rather

than forcing him or her to work—and possibly infecting others or extending their illness.

Employees want to stay with caring offices, and if you have this type of office, your employees will work to keep it thriving because they feel they are an integral part of it.

2. Fun at work

My office encourages team-building through games and friendly competition. We do things like have barbecues, pillow sack races, ball tosses, and rewards like cash or fun prizes. Not only does the team look forward to positive work surprises, but team members post and share the fun on social media. Our morning huddles start with a physical activity that gets the blood pumping and the body energized.

> *Encourage your team to become more cognizant of the patient as a whole person.*

3. Positive patient referrals

Besides delivering amazing patient care, we have to understand that patients come from all walks of life: rich, poor, gay, straight, religious, atheist, and so forth. Since we are in the service industry and they are paying for our services, we must respect their lifestyles. We may not agree with our patients, but we have to be neutral and not let our opinions get in the way of patient care. An example: A few years ago there was a legal effort in California to ban same-sex marriages. One of our colleagues put a sign in his waiting room showing his disapproval for same-sex marriage and urging people to vote against it. His office manager informed me (we were good friends) that he lost at least 50 patients because of that sign. Regardless of how you may feel, you are a health practitioner first and foremost, and satisfied patients refer others.

4. Larger profits

A great team will increase revenues in many ways:
- Better coordination of the daily schedule allows you to treat more patients without making them wait too long.
- Better patient management due to great communication between all departments. If your hygienist sees the need for a crown treatment and does the patient consultation, it is more likely that you can finish the treatment on the same day.
- Better rapport with a team member who has remained on your team longer results in higher case acceptance.
- Greater efficiency between doctors and assistants means that the room will set up perfectly by the assistant and the treatment will be done quickly and with great precision. I remember working in corporate dentistry and my assistant was fresh out of school. A simple filling took us over an hour because she had to get up from her chair at least five times to get something that she had forgotten.
- Greater efficiency in the amount of time the doctor spends with patients. When I go for an exam in the hygiene rooms, I'm in and out in less than three minutes. The hygienists do all the work, and I go in and double-check their findings and move on to the next patient.

Unfortunately, we can get very busy in running our offices and don't always have a chance to spend time to make our office a better place in which to work. Challenges such as these keep us occupied: the fluctuations in the schedule that will reduce revenue, the team who does not understand the doctor, not making the numbers, the business is slowing down, the lease is up and the rent will go up soon, and everything else under the sun. It is critical to make time for important business matters that will set a course of success for your office in the present and greatly impact it in the future.

IV. Great Companies, Great Cultures

Here are some examples of how companies have created a great company culture that helps them with great customer service:

> **They have to feel like they are part of a family that is growing and helping the world.**

Zappos.com is a 2 billion dollar company that sells shoes. Its team members go out of their way to ensure their customers are happy. Zappos offers new hires $2,000 to leave after the first week. It really wants to keep only people who truly want to stay. The company gives raises based on learned skills instead of office politics or the seniority of the employee.

Southwest Airlines has a loyal following like no other. I love them because they make it easier on me. Recently I booked a trip to Costa Rica through Delta Airlines and suddenly had to cancel it. Delta asked for a $200 change fee in spite of the fact that they occasionally have to offer $500 for someone to give up their seat because the airline oversold tickets. With Southwest when I change flights, there is a zero change fee. Not only is this better for the company's customers, but the employees who work for Southwest are also happier. In-flight joking is common, which gives travelers a stronger sense of connection and trust with the staff.

Twitter is another remarkable company with a great culture. They have team-oriented environments, free meals, and free yoga classes. They chose yoga because it calms the mind. Having mellow employees may seem counterproductive, but in the long run it makes them more productive.

V. Millennials in the Workforce

Today's employees are very different from previous generations of workers.

I'm astounded when I hear my patients say, "I'm retiring from working for the same company for 30 years." Yesteryear's employees would work for one or two employers for their entire careers before retiring. This is not the case now.

In today's fast-paced times, the average employee works for an employer for about five years or less. This means that all the effort and money put into the employee goes down the drain when the employee leaves. You have basically given the employee a free education, and now he or she is off to another job site. If you hire right and have a great culture that promotes your staff, chances are employees will stay with you for a longer time.

We are seeing a dramatic shift in employee-business relationships. Most of the employees that we will have in the next 10 years are called millennials. There are roughly 73 million millennials, born between 1982 and 1996. The millennials are used to fast-paced changes, efficiency in Internet and social media, and quick decision-making. Millennials often desire an environment that is constantly challenging, allowing them to grow and develop.

The millennial generation needs to fit in with their jobs, teams, and companies. They need a sense of purpose and strong group dynamics with opportunities for personal and professional growth. They tend to be educated and are constantly connected. They understand their options and seek employment that is fulfilling. They seek personal happiness in everything they do.

Here are some key points about millennials from a Gallup Poll:
- They are less politically involved and use the Internet over 70% of the time for news.
- They have a high rate of unemployment.
- They wait longer to get married and want to have fewer children.
- They like jobs that they see emotionally and behaviorally connected to them.
- They want to change the world for the better.

What does this means for us as employers? We need to meet or exceed their expectations or else they will not stay long with us. They have to feel like they are part of a family that is growing and helping the world. At the same time we also need to help our employees grow and become better.

2
Mastering Leadership Skills

People ask the difference between a leader and a boss. The leader leads, and the boss drives.
— Theodore Roosevelt

Are you a manager/boss, or are you a leader?

A manager/boss directs people in accomplishing tasks, and ensures that things get done. A leader shows people how to do things, so if the leader is not there, the people will still be able to do those things.

Companies like dental practices that have great leadership show it through their employees' commitment to excellence. When a company appreciates, educates, and motivates its team, its staff becomes content and does a better job. Revenues grow, securing a strong position for the company for future success.

Leading your team members is crucially important. With that being said, you need to trust your front office manager to manage your front office so that you can be free to lead and inspire your team. With enough practice, you will master the leadership skills you need to lead a successful dental practice.

To be a great leader of a successful dental practice, you must master certain skills:

I. Be Fluid

Bruce Lee said, "Be like water." Water adapts, taking the shape of the container that we put it into. A leader who is fluid, who is open to challenges and change, can better handle a variety of situations. We dentists deal with a lot of different situations, from patients who are not happy with the color of their gold crown (not yellow enough!), to a new hygienist who tells patients that they have great teeth and only need to floss three times a week. If we become more fluid, flexible leaders, we are then better able to handle different situations with different levels of empathy, strength, and courage. Sometimes we need to make an instant decision and at other times we need to wait to see how things develop.

> *Minor changes are a fact of life ... be open to them.*

II. Be Open-Minded

Life is constantly changing and so are dental innovations. Once you get used to something, you might get set in your ways and not want to try something new. But I can assure you, some things are worth changing. A good example is when I changed our dental resin system. For years we were using the dental resin system that I was trained for in dental school. The problem was that the brand of composite resin I was using couldn't be polished to a high shine. So, I did some research to find the best composite materials out there by talking to two highly-trained cosmetic dentists. They recommended a different brand and I tried it. It polished so well and the gloss was so amazing that even I couldn't tell what part was the tooth and what part was the filling! Minor changes are a fact of life—be open to them.

III. Invest Time in People

How do you build great relationships with people? Spend time with them. How do you have an outstanding dental office? Spend time with your team by providing them with great leadership! Time is the essence of everything.

IV. Focus on What's Important

There are very few things that are truly urgent in life and yet sometimes we make them urgent, creating stress for ourselves. Example: your hygiene schedule is full and your best hygienist calls in sick. Although it might be impossible to reach some patients to let them know about the cancellations, especially the first one scheduled, go ahead and do your best. Or possibly a patient is at the office and the lab still has not delivered the case like it promised yesterday. OK, apologize and move on with your day. If you take these problems personally you can really stress yourself out. Yes, there are urgent matters that need to be addressed, but they are not the same as having a patient in your dental chair who stops breathing—which is a real emergency!

V. Have a Game Plan

When issues arise, learn from them so that you will have a game plan to handle (or eliminate) those occurrences in the future. We cannot have a perfect day because we cannot possibly control everything. The only person we can control is ourselves, and even this is challenging at times, so stop trying to make everything perfect all the time.

In the case of a sick hygienist, for example, tell your staff to let your key office administrator know—the earlier the better. One of my key team members has access to our computers from her home. When one of my hygienists had a bad accident on a Sunday and could not come in the next day, we were able to reach the patients in time. From her home, my team member was able to reschedule all of the patients, and everything worked out on Monday. For our lab, we have a close relationship and have ironed out most of the past issues. When the lab says that they will bring in the case by a certain time, this usually happens—but we know from past experience that our removable lab is always late by 30 minutes, so we adjust our schedule to account for that lateness.

VI. Be Aware

See what is going on around you, and help if you are able. A couple of years ago, we were in need of a hygienist, and after eight months of looking we finally found one. She had a nice personality, was not set in her ways, was willing to learn, and had great people skills. But by week two I had noticed that her scrubs were all different colors and never matched, and she wore shoes that made her look like a high school student. We did not want this image to be the image of our office. So, I pulled her to the side, informed her of the situation, gave her $200 and asked her to please dress more professionally. I knew she was a recent graduate and didn't have much disposable income. After my gesture, she was in tears and told me that no doctor had ever helped her like this. From that moment on, she was always presentable.

VII. Know When to Say "No"

As a leader, sometimes you have to say "No" even though this may not make you popular. One of my long-term staff members (a hygienist) really wanted the office to be open the Monday after New Year's. New Year's Eve was on a Saturday that year, and we were closed the following Sunday and Monday. She really wanted the office to be open that Monday, but I believed that the majority of the patients would cancel or forget about their appointments right after the holidays, and I also wanted to give the team two days off in a row for working so hard the entire year. So, after thinking it over, I told her "No."

People will follow amazing leaders. Amazing leaders have a way of helping, promoting, and making the environment they are in a better place to work.

Thoughts and Ideas

3 Defining Job Positions

> *Coming together is a beginning. Keeping together is progress. Working together is success.*
>
> **Henry Ford**

All dental offices are composed of three major work areas, the front office or the business section, an area for the non-doctor clinical staff, and one for the doctors. Each area has a specific function and specific training needs; for example, we would not teach a doctor how to answer phone calls or teach the front office staff how to clean teeth. In a small, one-doctor practice, however, team members often do have job crossovers. For example, my front office handles treatment coordination, scheduling, and receptionist duties, but also takes X-rays.

I. Staff Roles

In order for employees to become good at what they do, they need to have a well-written game plan and the necessary training. Do you recall your first crown preparation in dental school? My prep took three hours and resembled Mount Fuji because of its excessive taper. We had been given a guide on how to prepare a tooth for a crown but no actual training. After training and much practice I can now prepare a tooth in less than 10 minutes with zero excessive taper.

If employees know what their job responsibilities are, they can work towards achieving and even surpassing them. Before meeting or hiring new employees we need to have a detailed list of expectations. For example, let's say we're hiring dental hygienists. Besides dental cleaning, what else will you require of them? Do they see the new patient first? Are they responsible for scheduling patients? What else do they need to work with you in order to help you build a better practice? What types of rewards will they get if they meet targets or challenges? Rewards and incentives can vary: bonuses, raises, appreciation, awards and recognition—anything you decide.

Giving the employees task directives allows your staff to work together smoothly, like cogs in a machine. Make all job descriptions available to all employees so that they are aware of what everyone should be doing during the day. By making employees self-sufficient you won't have to constantly look over their shoulders to make sure things are getting done. This frees up your time for other tasks like leadership, increasing doctor services, designing business productivities, and other highly productive managerial actions.

> *The main role of every employee is treating patients with kindness and empathy.*

In my office the main role of every employee is patient care - treating patients with kindness and empathy. We are there because of our patients, and we need to make sure that the needs of the patients are met. Thus, we include a section on being a caring person in each of our job descriptions. This is how great dental offices are made.

II. Punctuality and Social Media

Staying on time and not running late are very important. If your office is running late more than 5% of the time, then you need to change the schedule to account for this. For example, our hygienists are required to meet patients in the waiting room and walk them to their operatories. Once there, they can socialize with the patient and go over patient health. This should take about 5 to 10 minutes. Dental cleaning also includes interacting with patients to educate them, increase satisfaction, and get referrals.

We also use a social media module so that the patient and the team can increase our online awareness. The social media module includes asking for Facebook reviews, taking Facebook photos with the patient with fun signs that say, "I love my hygienist," and getting patient permission to share. The social media module only takes a few minutes and our patients love it. Afterwards, our hygienist walks the patient to the front office, schedules him or her for the next visit, and then goes back and gets ready for the next patient.

III. Employee Requirements

A job responsibility list is an important tool for the office.

All staff, everyone, must know all of the treatments that the office does, in order to be able to explain those treatments to patients. The why is more important than the how. Why do I need this crown? Why do I need this root canal?

Your staff should go beyond their normal job duties to help patients. If a patient needs water, bring them a bottle or glass of water. If a patient is cold, get them a blanket. If a patient needs to use the restroom, show them where it is by walking along the way with them. If a patient needs something that the office does not have, apologize and talk to the team leader. These small gestures make the office more patient-friendly.

Be professionally dressed (neat and clean scrubs, front office outfits, and doctor dress). Be conscious of your company culture in regards to makeup, hair, and clothing; patients have expectations when they come to an office. Have a detailed dress code to avoid any miscommunications. In my office, some staff wear makeup, others do not; both are acceptable as long as a professional appearance is maintained.

The front office has the first contact with a patient and should help the patient to feel cared for. So, when a patient telephones, the front desk has a duty to be pleasant and knowledgeable and assess the patient's needs.

Ideally, patient phone calls are handled in a systematic way:
- First, find out why the patient is calling.
- Second, determine how your office can help.
- Third, direct the patient to the quickest predetermined solution.

The front office must be able to overcome patient objections and answer patient questions, thoroughly check the insurance, and make appointments for patients to come in to the office. While helping patients, the front office must build and maintain a quality rapport. This must be done for any transaction to happen and for your office to keep a high standard of care and patient satisfaction. Your staff should greet walk-in patients, introduce them to the office, and talk with them in a comfortable way. Legal forms should be given to the patient and payment confirmed. The back office assistants should be introduced and gotten ready to go.

The front office staff confirms treatments. When explaining treatment to patients, staff should always describe the treatment in terms of how the treatment benefits the patient! For example, once in a while a patient will call our office and ask to move from a 3-month periodontal maintenance to every 6 months. Their concerns are reducing costs. The front office should be able to give reasons for maintaining the 3-month schedule other than "The hygienist says so," because the patient cannot understand how this answer benefits them, only that it hurts their pocketbooks. The correct answer communicates a direct benefit to the patient: "We want to help you keep your teeth for as long as possible. After gathering extensive data on gum disease and pus pockets, we know that the areas around your teeth have a higher tendency to hold more food and bacteria. This leads to the bone around your teeth being degraded and thus will cause your teeth to fall out and lead to other unsightly issues. By seeing us more often, we have greater success at removing the food and bacteria from around your teeth, allowing you to keep your teeth much longer."

Other duties of the front office include:
- Mastering dental insurance: know which companies pay how much for particular procedures and how to bill and collect from insurance companies.
- Showing mature etiquette when speaking with patients and dental insurance companies.
- Using proper terminology that brings positive results.

- Coordinating the daily schedule properly: full booking with room for emergencies and changes.
- Having a great attitude and being positive.
- Answering the phones properly and correctly.
- Being able to respond to the patient's concerns and questions.
- Giving estimates to existing patients correctly with all questions answered.
- Handling multiple phone lines and concurrently managing face-to-face patients.
- Presenting treatment plans in a logical and understandable way.
- Gauging the patient's emotions to elicit understanding of the treatment plan.
- Finishing their job in a timely manner.
- Asking for help if they fall behind.
- Knowing the goals of the office and working towards achieving them.

> *Having a good dental assistant who can listen and still get the job done is priceless.*

Office assistants take patients to the operatory and prepare them for the first step of treatment. This can take anywhere from 10-20 minutes. Assistants should know the benefits of different procedures. The doctor sometimes intimidates patients, so once the doctor leaves the room the patient may ask the dental assistant treatment questions. If the patient doesn't understand what the doctor is saying, the assistant should take the lead and become an "interpreter." The assistant should be able to explain the different treatments available to patients in an easy-to-understand way, avoiding technical dental terms that the average person doesn't understand. There's a higher chance of case acceptance if the dental assistant can tell the patients the benefits of a particular procedure.

Assistants should be positive, courteous, and empathetic - the patients look for the assistant's positive energy to get them through the treatment. Sometimes patients will talk about their problems - having a good dental assistant who can listen and still get the job done is priceless.

Assistants coordinate schedules with the back office, front office, doctors, and other staff and help manage patients. When a patient is passed from one staff member to the next, it should be done in a proper manner with introductions by name. Assistants should remember that they are taking care of the patient, and the doctor is there to finish and confirm the treatment. Once the doctor leaves the room it is the assistant's responsibility to finish patient customer service and walk them to the front office.

The dental hygienist's basic functions are to remove calculus and plaque. They should not cause pain to the patient no matter how deep the calculus is. If they see sub-gingival calculus they should talk to the patient about doing a limited deep cleaning at another time and explain their reasoning. They should make sure that the patient doesn't feel embarrassed and reassure them that what they have is normal, but let the patient know that the hygienist will need to take extra precautions for their comfort. The hygienist should talk to the patients about existing treatment plans and other areas of the mouth that need work. If they see broken teeth, cracked fillings, severe discoloration, or anything else that matters, they should mention it to the patient and the doctor during the examination.

Great dental hygienists are very important. They help build rapport with the patients, talk about existing and possible treatment, and reduce the amount of time doctors spend in the room. There has been a big shift in the role of dental hygienists in our field. The role of the hygienists has become more and more about educating patients in treatment. In my office, when the dental hygienist sees children with crooked teeth she talks to parents about braces. If a patient has gaps in his or her teeth, she talks to the patient about dental implants. Hygienists are doing the work for us so that we doctors can focus on larger treatments.

The doctor has the sole responsibility for the entire office, doing everything at the master or specialist level. For example, placing brackets puts you at the orthodontist level. It is critical that you get extensive training and know your stuff. It's also beneficial to offer many procedures to stay competitive and profitable. The doctor also has to be a master of marketing, a human resource director, CEO, CFO, mentor, and occasionally act as a parent. As the doctor, owner, and team leader, you have a lot of responsibilities. You have a unique position, but with a solid task list and delegation you can have a business run smoothly.

> *You are a doctor, and because of that, you must appear invincible.*

Doctors' responsibilities include:
- Screening for oral cancer.
- Mastering the treatments performed on patients.
- Learning to talk to patients in a realistic way that they can understand. They don't understand a tooth needs a root canal because there is a shadow on the x-ray; however, they do understand when you say the tooth is dead and causing an infection.
- Leading your team by example and with open communication.
- Learning to manage your business so that the flow is maintained and the drama is kept to a minimum.

- Following future forecasts and studying how they will affect your business directly. Use Google options.
- Bringing in new procedures that will benefit your patients and increase revenue. Make a plan to bring in a new procedure every few years.
- Knowing what your most and least profitable procedures are.
- Encouraging the procedures you like and discouraging the ones you would prefer not to do. Raise fees on the complicated procedures you feel take the most time and energy.
- Coming to work with a positive outlook on life. Your team and patients look up to you. If you're having a bad day it will affect morale and possibly cost you a patient or two. You are a doctor, and because of that, you must appear invincible.

Positions That Need Improvement

Front Office

POOR   1 • 2 • 3 • 4 • 5 • 6 • 7 • 8 • 9 • 10   GREAT

Areas of Improvement

_____

_____

_____

Dental Assistant

POOR   1 • 2 • 3 • 4 • 5 • 6 • 7 • 8 • 9 • 10   GREAT

Areas of Improvement

_____

_____

_____

Positions That Need Improvement

Dental Hygienist
POOR   1 • 2 • 3 • 4 • 5 • 6 • 7 • 8 • 9 • 10   GREAT
Areas of Improvement

_____
_____
_____

Dentist
POOR   1 • 2 • 3 • 4 • 5 • 6 • 7 • 8 • 9 • 10   GREAT
Areas of Improvement

_____
_____
_____

Position _____
POOR   1 • 2 • 3 • 4 • 5 • 6 • 7 • 8 • 9 • 10   GREAT
Areas of Improvement

_____
_____
_____

Position _____
POOR   1 • 2 • 3 • 4 • 5 • 6 • 7 • 8 • 9 • 10   GREAT
Areas of Improvement

_____
_____
_____

4 Crafting the Optimal Help-Wanted Ad

Alone we can do so little, together we can do so much.

Helen Keller

I. The Impactful Ad

Good help wanted ads are impactful and do the most important thing: find us the right candidate for the opening. We cannot expect to find a great candidate if we don't put time and effort into crafting a strong and straightforward advertisement. Before you write the specifics, it's important to think of what you honestly want from the employee. With the right ad, expect to get many applicants. The truth is, 90% of the applicants who apply for your job won't be qualified or a good fit for your office culture. Do not be misleading; employees expect the position you are selling. Corporate dental offices tend to offer "great opportunities for advancement" yet they pay their employees minimum wage and put a tremendous workload on them, so naturally employees don't stay long. Talk about the amazing people that comprise your dental office and the insurances that you accept. Insurance is key because people in the dental field know that certain kinds of insurance indicates the office is run on a very tight budget and may have a high turnover rate.

II. What to Include

Now that you have talked about the office, you want to describe the specific criteria that you are looking for. For example, if your dental office is a Pediatric, Orthodontic, or any other specialty field, customize your ad accordingly.

Include software technology and specific equipment such as the digital x-ray system you're using, the dental operating software that you have, if you use same-day crowns or take impressions, and how much interaction is needed with patients.

> *Grow and learn with a caring doctor, a great team, in a fun and exciting environment.*

Key elements:
- What to expect
- A description of your office and practice
- Why you are seeking another staff member
- Your company culture or philosophy (you must establish this beforehand)
- Benefits and bonuses
- Education or training offered
- Education or training required for the position
- Work requirements: hours and days
- Appearance or professional manner expectation
- Personality expectations
- Travel, reception, and other additional office tasks

Another challenge that I've experienced in the past is when a dental office is too far from the city and gets low job applicant numbers. The most important thing, however, is to hire on behavior and great attitude.

Enthusiastic Team Member Wanted
(Sample of one of our ads.)

Great fee-for-service dental office is looking for an amazing team member! We have long-term staff with very low turnover. The staff member that you're replacing has been with us for years and is going back to school to further her education. We are an office like no other and expect top quality team members. We are looking for an energetic person who's willing to learn and grow. We offer a great PTO plan, bonuses, and extra training in patient care, customer service, and team dynamics. Some of our past training sessions were in Miami, Las Vegas, Los Angeles, and many other fun places. We require a minimum of three years of experience in the dental field (two years in a general dental office), professional appearance in dress and hygiene, and good communication skills. You must be experienced with Dentrix, have extensive knowledge about dental insurance, be able to make chair-side temporary crowns and bridges, and be comfortable with helping the doctor place implants. The position requires you to work Monday through Friday 8am-5pm, with occasional Fridays off. Our team training also requires some weekend education courses. We are focused on great patient care and we empower our employees by educating them, giving them autonomy, and encouraging them to become great. We have regular team meetings so the right candidate will need to be open to change and presenting to the group.

IV. Targeting the Candidates

Here are some questions to think about when somebody is responding to a help wanted ad:
- Why are they looking for work after working somewhere else?
- Will they leave my office in a short amount of time to find a better place to work?
- If they don't have a job right now, why aren't they working?
- Are they a terrible employee?
- Can they keep up with modern work requirements to secure a job?

Good employees with great work ethics are always working. These are the types of employees that you want. In order for you to attract them, your office must offer a better workplace than their current job does. I don't mean just in terms of income; I mean the whole package: the ability to grow and learn, being with a team and a caring doctor, and being in a fun and exciting environment.

99 90% of the applicants who apply for your job won't be qualified or a good fit for your office culture.

My best and longest-term team members came from the following situations:
- They had recently relocated to the area.
- Their office closed down, or sold, or their hours were being cut (we found three amazing team members this way).

Remember, there are a lot of possibilities for great people and your task is to attract them. And, if you provide a great place to work, keep them motivated, and strive for their happiness you won't have to fight a high turnover rate.

V. Employment Ad Venues

Years ago if you wanted to find an employee there were only two options: a poster or newspaper ad. I remember taking out an ad in the newspaper and being charged $150 to run a classified post for one week. That is not the case any longer. Here are my suggested candidate avenues:

Craigslist: By far the best source because it's economical (around $35, with some locations free) and you get results.

Local dental staffing services: Great because you do not initially hire the employee so you can give the employee a chance to see if they're a good fit. The screening has been already done by the agency, so the only thing that you want to find out is whether or not this person will fit in your culture. The drawback is the heavy expense you will pay. Expect to pay around 20% more to hire, but it's actually worth it if you find the right employee.

Local district dental society newsletters: Not all people in the dental field go to these sources but they work well if you're seeking an employee who has been in the dental field for many years. When I put ads in these newsletters I often get employees who are close to retirement.

Headhunting: While this may be taboo in our field, it's still fairly common for a reason: unhappy employees are looking for ways to improve their lives, so if you provide the best work environment you will be able to pick from the best candidates. If their current job isn't allowing them to grow and develop then by all means they have a right to leave.

Referrals: The dental community is small and people in the field know about other offices. Employees know one another from school, conferences, educational meetings, Facebook, and social events. If your office is well-known and respected in the community, you won't have problems in filling vacancies.

<u>**Most Important Points
for Your Optimal Ad**</u>

1 _____

2 _____

3 _____

4 _____

5 _____

6 _____

7 _____

5 Before the Interview

Fortune favors the prepared mind.

Louis Pasteur

Up to this point we have done a tremendous amount of work. We've made sure there's dedicated leadership with a focus on having an office game plan, patient care, and high employee satisfaction. We have a great and thorough job responsibility list for every position, and we have put out an amazing help wanted ad. Now what?

I. Don't Rush!

The lack of a needed employee can wreak havoc on scheduling and patient care. Most of the time, the person in charge of hiring gets excited about the first few applicants and wants to fill the opening as soon as possible. It's tempting to fill a position quickly so that the business can operate at normal levels and profits will go back up. Yet if we rush into things and don't do our research on potential candidates we can bring in elements that are worse than having a missing team member. Having the wrong employee is guaranteed to cause a lot of problems: lack of teamwork, internal drama, someone having to take the time to deal with the bad employee, potential harm to patients, destructive online reviews, and overall loss of productivity.

So before we begin the arduous task of rifling through applicants we need to delegate interview tasks and set up the appropriate schedule.

Answer the following questions:
- Who is the first contact person for the applicants?
- What criteria should we use to filter the applicants?
- What days do you set aside for group interviews?
- What is the best way to contact your office: email or phone number?
- Do you have a dedicated email/phone number for applicants?

II. Previewing and Resumes

Resumes are the introductory page to a potential candidate. We have no way of knowing about their qualifications or personality beforehand; our first given source is their resume.

Don't let great presentations, graphics or photos dazzle you. Get to the meat of the resume.

Your job as a business owner is to break down the resumes into their most crucial parts and make an assessment about the candidate. In my experience, 80% of the resumes that we receive don't fit our office criteria, so we throw those away. For example, in asking for a registered dental assistant we have also received resumes from cashiers, restaurant workers, and many other applicants with no dental experience. The employment market is confusing for many people. I can't fault them for hoping for a better job but regardless, it does waste time.

When you're looking at resumes, don't get dazzled by the great templates, great presentation, high-impact graphics, the candidate's photo, or other superficial things. Those things are fun to look at, yet you want to get to the meat of the resume.

III. The Five Steps to Review a Resume

1. First Glance

Spend 10 seconds reviewing an initial resume. I want to make sure that the candidate is qualified for the dental field. We have had candidates in the past that finished dental assisting school yet worked in non-dental fields like real estate or restaurants for extended time periods. The problem is that these candidates have lost, forgotten, and/or have never used the skills they were trained in. Academic education is good for the basics but to have a stellar office we need to seek professionals with relevant field experience. The applicants who clear step one go to step two.

2. Work History

Glance through work history. If candidates have short spans of work history chances are they will stay with us only a short time. One time we hired a great employee with the majority of her work history lasting between one and two years. I thought maybe our office would make a difference for her, but ultimately she stayed with us for only about a year and a half. So all the time, energy, and educational money we invested in this employee was gone with her when she left.

3. The Licensing Board

Do a quick review from the licensing board. Anyone with some kind of registered training will have a record of their information on the board's website. The main reason why I check their record is to make sure that the license is not suspended. We had a dental hygienist applicant who seemed qualified but did not put her license number on her resume. After a little research we discovered that the candidate had a suspended license. As doctors and owners we are obligated to follow licensing laws. If we have an employee with a suspended license we get in big trouble if something happens. Not only we are allowing a non-licensed employee to perform licensed work, which is illegal, but we are also opening ourselves to lawsuits and the end of our trustworthy reputation.

4. Social Media and Web Search

Use social media and search engines. I also dig deeper into who they are in a public setting. With today's technology and online search capabilities our business is constantly being scrutinized, so it's important to make sure any candidate is free from scandal. If you see lots of photos of highly questionable behavior, comments about rudeness and negativity, or the candidate portraying themselves as a predator, the chances are high that that same behavior will come to the work site. Because we are in the service industry, as well as the public eye, we must be vigilant as to what our team members are bringing to our offices. We need to protect our patients, our office, our team, and ourselves from those who would do us harm, even if unintentionally.

5. Contact Employers

Finally, look at the candidate's last three employers. A quick search of the office or doctors' names will result in a plethora of information. I view the employers' websites and see what kind of business models they have. Before calling, I check to see if the candidate is currently working at their last place; I don't call current employers so the candidate won't get into trouble.

Some owners will understand your inquiry and give more than you ask for but having a good question list is essential.

In phone calls with past employers:
- Get as much information about the work ethics of this employee from the last employer, so ask open-ended questions.
- Use a qualifying statement like, "Hi, my name is Dr. Ike Rahimi. We received a resume from a candidate who used to work for you. May I take a few minutes of your time to ask you a few questions?"
- Ask about the candidate's interaction with patients and other staff, punctuality, being a team player, or anything else that made them stand out.
- Be polite and sincere. Remember, if the candidate was horrible, the last employer will hint that to you so that you don't hire them.

Your job as the employer is to weed out the resumes while wasting as little of your time as possible. If you are doing it, it's your time. If someone else is doing it, you are paying that person's wages. There is no going around this task but reduce the time spent in this phase as much as possible.

Consider What Questions to Ask Previous Employers

1 _____

2 _____

3 _____

4 _____

5 _____

6 _____

7 _____

8 _____

9 _____

10 _____

11 _____

Conducting the Interview

Talent wins games, but teamwork and intelligence wins championships.

Michael Jordan

There are many different approaches to interviewing prospective employees. I prefer to conduct a behavioral interview.

I. Behavioral Interviews

Traditional interviews are where the employer asks the potential employee a bunch of prepared questions. Prospective employees can be really good at answering questions and still not function properly in certain work environments. One strong filter is the use of behavioral interviews.

Behavioral interviews assess the competence, personality, and social skills of the candidate. As you look for great team members, ask appropriate questions and listen to how they said they behaved in the past in given situations. Behavioral interviews are more predictive of future on-the-job behavior than traditional interviews. If the person acted or reacted poorly or well in the past, chances are they will act or react the same way in the future.

Ask open-ended behavioral questions, such as:
- "Imagine you had a long week and one your co-workers is sick on a Friday. Everyone's tired and the mood is down. How would you work that day and how would you cheer up your team members?"
- "Tell me about a challenging day at your last job and how you overcame the challenge."
- "If a customer is truly angry or unhappy about a particular product or service, what kind of methods can you use to reduce their anxiety? Please elaborate on at least three methods."

II. Leadership and Mediation

Ask the candidate what he or she would do in certain conflict scenarios. For example: a patient is not happy with the color of their crown; a patient came in today for her appointment but it's tomorrow; or two employees don't seem to get along. You want to make sure that the candidate is able to deal with issues in the workplace.

> *When someone admits failure, listen without judging them. They are taking responsibility for their actions.*

Inquire about their attitude towards failure and growth. Have them discuss with you three times they failed and what they learned from them. We all have failures and if a candidate says they never fail, take that as a giant red flag. Failure is part of developing and growing as a professional and as a well-adjusted, mature person. Some people blame others for their problems and never own their issues and thus never learn and grow. Years ago, I had an assistant who never owned her mistakes—it was always someone else's fault, and the office atmosphere was always very tense. After a short time she left and the office atmosphere became a lot better.

When someone admits failure, we should listen to their admissions without judging them: they are human, and they are taking responsibility for their actions.

III. Team Players and Problem Solvers

Other questions you can ask are, "If a patient comes in and doesn't want to start a conversation, yet they have issues in their mouth, how would you overcome the situation? How would you communicate to the patient how important it is that they get the problem taken care of?" As the candidate answers these questions you want to be aware of how they answer. Are they comfortable with problem solving? Or are they only there for a potential paycheck? Before you move on to the working interview, go through the interactive questions to give you an idea of how the candidate behaves in certain situations.

Up to this point we have talked about how to interview in a way that brings out the behavioral actions of the new team members. Now let's talk about the actual interview process.

IV. The Four Types of Dental Interviews

1. The Phone Interview (15-20 Minutes)

Phone interviews are a relatively new idea for small businesses, though larger businesses have been doing this for quite some time. The reason why phone interviews are popular is that you can minimize the time wasted on your search to find a potential candidate. Phone interviews take little time and you can still reduce the number of people that you will take to the next step. A nice thing about a phone interview is that you can do it after hours when it's more convenient for you or your office manager. I once did a phone interview at 8:30 pm. We were looking to fill a hygiene position and this candidate was working during the day. We played a lot of phone tag but finally got a hold of each other late in the evening.

> *Just as fitness trainers have to look presentable and be fit, so must the members of your team ... and so must their teeth.*

Comparing phone interview costs to one-on-one interview costs: Years ago we were looking for a dental hygienist. We put out a great ad, got 50 resumes and picked 15 for a closer look. Here is the in-person office cost associated with interviewing for that position: each office interview of 30-45 minutes cost about $100 in staff and doctor time, so the total cost of interviewing all 15 candidates was approximately $1,500. If interviewing 15 candidates costs our office $1,500 (at a minimum), and at the end we only have a spot for one person, why are we wasting so much money on in-person interviews when we can reduce the 15 candidates to just a handful through a phone call? Further, the most profitable team member (the lead doctor) doesn't have to handle the call if you have someone else in charge of the hiring process. In most small dental offices, however, the doctor is in charge of this duty.

2. The One-on-One Interview (30 Minutes)

Remember that the candidate is nervous and so you'll want to help them relax so they can feel comfortable. Tell them, "It's OK to be nervous. We have plenty of time for this meeting and you will do great."

Does the candidate reflect the position? In other words, is the candidate on time and prepared (clean, professionally dressed for that job)?

Appearances matter. We have to look presentable in our profession and if we don't, then patients don't take us seriously.

I used to go to a nearby gym and was thinking about getting a personal trainer. My goal was to build muscle mass and look thinner. The first male trainer I had was 40% overweight. I switched because I figured if he could not lose weight, how could he help me? The second trainer was a very skinny female who could barely lift 25 pounds. Since I did not want to be that skinny, I left that trainer. The third one was a beer-drinking divorced father who complained about the lack of money he was making; obviously he did not work well for me. Now I have found a perfect fit: a young woman that competes in various sports, has muscles, is fit, and knows about proper diet. Just as fitness trainers have to look presentable and be fit, so must the members of your team—and their teeth are of particular importance.

Do they have nice teeth? What kind of an image do you send your patients if members of your team have horrible and/or missing teeth? I'm sure you would want to fix their teeth, but what if they don't want it? Years ago we hired a great hygienist for some temporary work but her teeth were really misaligned. I offered to fix that for her but she refused. The patients liked her because of her great personality but she never convinced a single patient to get his or her own crooked teeth fixed.

Be aware of how your patients might react to a potential team member's appearance. Some time ago we were looking for a dental assistant and found what looked like the perfect fit. During the in-person interview my team noticed that she had tattoos on her neck and hands. This person had all the right fittings for the position but my office serves older, more conservative patients. Unless we had a position involving no face-to-face contact with patients—we didn't—we simply could not hire this person, in spite of her qualifications.

```
3. The Team Interview (30 Minutes)
```

I believe this is the most important part of an interview because you get experienced team members helping assess the candidate. Before the candidate actually gets in front of your group, get your team together and have a set game plan for the discussion. Use open-ended and conversational inquiries to encourage a team atmosphere. Another great benefit of having your whole team involved is ensuring the new person is trained well. It's important to get a jump-start so they can fit into the work culture as quickly and comfortably as possible. By delegating responsibility we are able to ensure that each team member becomes invested and, in the case of hiring errors, no one person is to blame.

4. The Working Interview (Full Day)

Working interviews are amazing because you can actually see the potential employee on the job.

Here are key things to watch for while observing them in their potential employment:
- How is their comfort level being in a new environment?
- Are they coping in a positive way that allows them to learn more?
- Are they resistant and awkward?
- How is their interaction with other team members?
- Do they respect group efforts and understand hierarchy?
- Can they see themselves meshing into a long-term work relationship?
- Do they give credit and respond thankfully? The worst thing we can do is hire someone who isn't a team player and wants all the credit.
- How are their interactions with patients? We have to keep in mind that we are here because of our patients; some patients may become stressed from knowing a new person is working them on.
- Professional appearance is important. Improper dress (according to your dress code) or poor hygiene doesn't bode well.

V. The Final Review

Ask your team members about their assessment of the potential new candidate. Hiring the right person takes time and energy. There are lots of steps that we need to follow to maximize our chances of getting the right team member and not allowing the wrong team member to slip in. A bad hire will cost the office money and frustration. Take your time and don't rush the process. It's perfectly all right to reduce your patient schedule while you are searching for the right person.

What Key Traits Will Help Any Candidate Join the Team?

1 _____

2 _____

3 _____

4 _____

5 _____

6 _____

7 _____

7 Introducing the Newest Team Member

Leadership and learning are indispensable to each other.

John F. Kennedy

Now the real work begins!

Since every dental office is different, it's up to us to help the new employee to connect with, and blend into, our culture. On average it takes almost one year for new employees to fully assimilate into your practice.

I. Encourage Acceptance

Patient satisfaction is our priority and new team members can affect the patient experience. There will be questions from patients about the new person, and they may need to see him or her a few times before feeling comfortable. It takes from 3-5 interactions for a patient to feel comfortable with a new employee. This means that patients who come in every 6 months will need 1-2 years to gain trust and rapport with the new employee. There is a direct correlation between having good case acceptance rates and long-term employees; patients enjoy seeing familiar faces.

II. The New Employee's Life Story

Have the employee write a short life synopsis that includes their education, family, hobbies, and anything else that is important to him or her (but is not sensitive or private). Share a printed copy with the entire team so that they can be aware and interact with patients accordingly. Make sure all team members are on the same page and deliver a great message to evoke the patients' positive and friendly emotions.

III. Employee Manual

The state in which you practice will determine the bulk of what to include in your employee manual. The best resource is your local dental society or state dental association to get a great template to start your employee manual.

> *Having good case acceptance rates and long-term employees are directly related ... patients enjoy seeing familiar faces.*

The employee manual template that you get should have areas that you will adjust based on your office protocol. For example, in my office the front office staff can have long manicured nails while anyone who works in a patient's mouth cannot have nails longer than 5mm and can use only clear nail polish. We also don't allow unnatural hair color (pink, purple, and so on). By setting the standard, you will communicate to the employee how the office flow works.

IV. Your Employees are Your Best Trainers

Job shadowing is great and gives a better interaction experience. This way they learn great habits to emulate and follow. This is critical when talking to patients. If your office allows for extra time if the patient wants to stay for treatment, then this needs to be communicated to the new hire. We know that all dental offices do not run the same. Some offices never squeeze in patients; many established offices have doctors who want to work less and don't want to push themselves to exhaustion.

The sink or swim approach does not work. New hires need to be properly trained in a friendly and respectful way. If we are forceful and treat them poorly they are more likely to treat your patients and other team members in the same fashion. Or even worse—they may feel that they don't belong and end up leaving.

Many years ago when I was a student at the University of California at Davis, I enrolled in an internship program dealing with OSHA guidelines. My duties included going to department heads and reviewing their OSHA logs to make sure that they were up to date. When I went to my first day of training, I received just one hour of instruction and was given a large binder to go home and read (which was full of laws I didn't understand). The woman in charge gave me a list of different department heads I should contact and visit but she wasn't going to be able to mentor me as she was going on vacation. Visiting the different departments was awkward in the extreme; I felt unprepared due to the lack of training. I quit what could've been a great opportunity because of a lack of guidance and leadership.

V. In the Beginning, Be a Guide

When we hire somebody new we explain to the new member that in our office, the skills he or she previously acquired may not be applicable. Years of experience in one dental office may not be transferable to the new office. Doctors need to manage company culture through discussions and straightforward conversations. Explain to the new hire that we are a unique and amazing dental office with our own dental culture. Listen for incorrect information between staff and patients. Ensure that new employees understand that they aren't in trouble and that constructive criticism is important to keep high standards. A great team doesn't develop by chance but rather because they are actively involved individuals and know how to give stellar patient care. Reassure the new member that everyone on the team had to learn and make personal efforts for months before settling in.

> *The sink or swim approach does not work ... show them, train them, help them succeed.*

It takes almost one year for the new hire to fully assimilate into a typical dental office, and it takes the entire team to guide a team member, so if the new hire has any challenges, these should be communicated. In some offices the line of communication does not exist and there is a lot of bottled-up frustration. Talking about difficult issues frees us and we also feel a lot better. Not only that, but by sharing a problem with a group, members can put their minds together to solve an issue. Every office is different - they take different insurances, they have a different philosophy of practicing dentistry, and the doctor(s) may be in different stages of their careers. We have to communicate these elements to the new hire.

VI. Patient Care Matters to Every Employee

For years the dental field was stable, and we didn't have to wear so many different hats; the recession changed that. The entire office has an active role in making sure that we stay busy. As the leader you have to make sure that the new employee understands a patient-driven business. We face competition from corporate dentistry and other dental offices. Patients have lots of options and if you give them a reason to, they will leave. Therefore, we have to work diligently to make sure our patients like us so that the entire staff will have enough hours to work and can pay their bills. New employees need to understand how office revenues are earned: we are rendering services to people and in return they are giving us their hard-earned money. Without patients we would not be here! The fewer insurance providers you support, the higher your patient care and satisfaction must be. Since the patients are paying the difference out of their pocket, they need a reason to stay with you. Thus, your team must have continual training in all phases of dentistry in order to have a better understanding of how to treat a patient right.

VII. Don't Forget About the Fun Stuff

In our office we throw a yearly patient appreciation party, get involved in charity organizations, donate to many fulfilling and local causes, and sometimes do pro bono cases for loyal patients who are going through tough times.

We have taken some fun trips to Miami, the Bahamas, Los Angeles, Disney World, and Las Vegas. Plus, we do regular office barbecues and other events. All these little things make the office a better place and team members want to stay and help me succeed.

VIII. Make Sure They Know: Change is Constant

My office culture is one that embraces growth and adaptation. I remind my team that the only thing constant is change and that we have to be flexible to provide enough work for all team members to get enough hours. When the recession of 2008 happened, my office went from being open four days a week to being open just two and a half days a week. This was horrible because the employees who used to work 35 hours a week suddenly were only working 25 hours a week. We were able to turn this around through trial and error by adjusting our office to fit the needs of our patients. Many people tend to like things to be consistent. If you have children or pets then you become adaptive to their habits and schedules. My little Yorkie dog wants to play ball in the morning and sleep by early evening. She is confused by changes in her schedule. The same principle applies to people. If you get people used to a schedule it can be detrimental to making big changes. Use minor changes on a regular basis such as alternating members leading group meetings, end-of-year events, and different ways of interacting with the patients. This way, people are used to and are open to bigger change when the time comes for it. Remember that our field is always changing and we need to be fluid and flexible with changes instead of going against them.

8 Training and Education

> *Educating the mind without educating the heart is no education at all.*
>
> — Aristotle

There's nothing more important than training and educating your team members. If you have a winning team and bring a new person on board, chances are high that the new person may not have been trained in excellent customer service. Train them. Show them what you want them to do, and model how you expect them to behave.

I used to go to about 100 hours of continuing education a year, learning how to do better root canals, place dental implants, and other procedures. I would purchase new equipment and spend countless hours on planning new procedures. I would spend weekends learning how to do a new procedure like a gingival graft and then announce on the following Monday that we were now doing gingival grafts. My team would look at me funny because they had no idea what the heck I was talking about. I was excited about the new procedures, yet as weeks passed I didn't get any patients interested in the grafts. Looking back, I unintentionally created a disconnect between what I was doing and what my team understood. I wasn't being a good team player.

After much frustration, I decided to take my team to these courses. It was hard to justify the price at the beginning (the cost may have been upwards of $20,000 with a full team attending) but the payoff was well worth it.

Here's what educating my staff did for my office:
- They know the procedures and can discuss them with patients.
- They know my preferences and timing.
- We work as a fluid team because they know the full scope of what will be done.
- By going to educational meetings together, we build stronger bonds and learn to co-operate better.
- Training gives them something to look forward to when traveling to an exciting place.

By educating the new team member you are helping them grow and develop within your team. Employees working within a system of advancement through education will develop overall betterment for the entire office. Empowered people love being part of a great team and do their best to stay aboard. There is nothing worse than seeing a great employee working for an employer who does not allow them to grow.

9

A Full Employee Checklist

If you're managing people rather than leading them and tracking time rather than results, you've already lost.
        Dr. Karan M. Pai

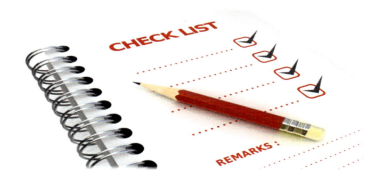

A Full Employee Checklist

Experience and Skills   ☐ YES • ☐ NO

_____

_____

POOR   1 • 2 • 3 • 4 • 5 • 6 • 7 • 8 • 9 • 10   GREAT

Typing (pro level is 65-75 wpm)   ☐ YES • ☐ NO

_____

_____

POOR   1 • 2 • 3 • 4 • 5 • 6 • 7 • 8 • 9 • 10   GREAT

Answering phones   ☐ YES • ☐ NO

_____

_____

POOR   1 • 2 • 3 • 4 • 5 • 6 • 7 • 8 • 9 • 10   GREAT

Confirming appointments   ☐ YES • ☐ NO

_____

_____

POOR   1 • 2 • 3 • 4 • 5 • 6 • 7 • 8 • 9 • 10   GREAT

Confirming appointments online   ☐ YES • ☐ NO

_____

_____

POOR   1 • 2 • 3 • 4 • 5 • 6 • 7 • 8 • 9 • 10   GREAT

A Full Employee Checklist

Checking out patients ☐ YES • ☐ NO

_____
_____

POOR   1 • 2 • 3 • 4 • 5 • 6 • 7 • 8 • 9 • 10   GREAT

Scheduling appointments ☐ YES • ☐ NO

_____
_____

POOR   1 • 2 • 3 • 4 • 5 • 6 • 7 • 8 • 9 • 10   GREAT

Collections / asking for money ☐ YES • ☐ NO

_____
_____

POOR   1 • 2 • 3 • 4 • 5 • 6 • 7 • 8 • 9 • 10   GREAT

Account collections ☐ YES • ☐ NO

_____
_____

POOR   1 • 2 • 3 • 4 • 5 • 6 • 7 • 8 • 9 • 10   GREAT

Treatment presentations ☐ YES • ☐ NO

_____
_____

POOR   1 • 2 • 3 • 4 • 5 • 6 • 7 • 8 • 9 • 10   GREAT

A Full Employee Checklist

Dental terminology for procedures ☐ YES • ☐ NO

_____

_____

POOR   1 • 2 • 3 • 4 • 5 • 6 • 7 • 8 • 9 • 10   GREAT

Dental insurance knowledge ☐ YES • ☐ NO

_____

_____

POOR   1 • 2 • 3 • 4 • 5 • 6 • 7 • 8 • 9 • 10   GREAT

Insurance claim processing ☐ YES • ☐ NO

_____

_____

POOR   1 • 2 • 3 • 4 • 5 • 6 • 7 • 8 • 9 • 10   GREAT

Pre-authorization processing ☐ YES • ☐ NO

_____

_____

POOR   1 • 2 • 3 • 4 • 5 • 6 • 7 • 8 • 9 • 10   GREAT

Office dental software ☐ YES • ☐ NO

_____

_____

POOR   1 • 2 • 3 • 4 • 5 • 6 • 7 • 8 • 9 • 10   GREAT

A Full Employee Checklist

Basic office software ☐ YES • ☐ NO

_____
_____

POOR   1 • 2 • 3 • 4 • 5 • 6 • 7 • 8 • 9 • 10   GREAT

Social media marketing knowledge ☐ YES • ☐ NO

_____
_____

POOR   1 • 2 • 3 • 4 • 5 • 6 • 7 • 8 • 9 • 10   GREAT

Computer knowledge ☐ YES • ☐ NO

_____
_____

POOR   1 • 2 • 3 • 4 • 5 • 6 • 7 • 8 • 9 • 10   GREAT

Addressing correspondence ☐ YES • ☐ NO

_____
_____

POOR   1 • 2 • 3 • 4 • 5 • 6 • 7 • 8 • 9 • 10   GREAT

CPR training ☐ YES • ☐ NO

_____
_____

POOR   1 • 2 • 3 • 4 • 5 • 6 • 7 • 8 • 9 • 10   GREAT

A Full Employee Checklist

Any other skills to be that may apply to this position

_____
_____
_____
_____
_____
_____
_____
_____
_____
_____
_____
_____
_____
_____
_____
_____
_____
_____
_____
_____
_____
_____

10

Questions

Every

Dental Office

Must Answer

♦

A Worksheet

What is the fundamental purpose of our business?

To build a solid foundation for a successful business, a well-written mission statement and vision are essential. A mission statement describes what a company does now; a vision statement outlines what a company wants to be in the future. The mission statement should define the fundamental purpose and values of our company, and the vision should be something for our company to aspire to. If we don't live up to our mission statement (why and how well we do what we do now), we will not achieve our vision (what we want to be in the future).

In my opinion, our current status is

POOR　　1 • 2 • 3 • 4 • 5 • 6 • 7 • 8 • 9 • 10　　GREAT

Mission Statement Thoughts and Ideas

_____
_____
_____
_____
_____
_____
_____
_____
_____

Questions to Consider

A. Do we have a well-written mission statement and vision?
☐ YES • ☐ NO

B. Is our team clear on the fundamental purpose of our dental office?
☐ YES • ☐ NO

C. Does our team believe in our purpose?
☐ YES • ☐ NO

D. Do the actions of our team truly reflect our purpose?
☐ YES • ☐ NO

E. Do we review our office's mission statement and vision on a periodic basis to be sure they are still relevant to the ever-changing marketplace?
☐ YES • ☐ NO

Vision Statement Thoughts and Ideas

_____
_____
_____
_____
_____
_____
_____
_____
_____
_____

What is the culture of our dental office?

If we don't clearly define the culture of our dental office, others will define it in their terms. Employees, patients, and competitors will react according to their perception of the principles and values we appear to live by. It is preferable to define our own core values, which in turn shape our office culture. There should be no doubt in the minds of our employees, patients, and competitors what our values and principles are. The key is to define those values and, more importantly, exemplify them by our actions.

In my opinion, our current status is

POOR   1 • 2 • 3 • 4 • 5 • 6 • 7 • 8 • 9 • 10   GREAT

5 Values Our Culture Should Reflect

1 _____

_____

_____

2 _____

_____

_____

3 _____

_____

_____

Questions to Consider

A. Do we have a functional culture in our office?
☐ YES • ☐ NO

B. Does every person in the office know and understand what our core values are?
☐ YES • ☐ NO

C. Can we identify 10 core values that we live by?
☐ YES • ☐ NO

5 Values Our Culture Should Reflect

4 _____

_____

_____

_____

5 _____

_____

_____

_____

Is our strategic position aligned with the patients' needs and wants?

In today's highly competitive, fast-paced, global marketplace we must constantly evaluate our strategic positioning. What worked in the past (last month) may not work in the future (next week). If we are going to win the 100-yard hurdles race, we have to find a way to clear the hurdles efficiently and not let them slow us down. Our ability to adapt our strategy to new challenges and opportunities will ultimately determine our destiny.

In my opinion, our current status is
POOR 1 • 2 • 3 • 4 • 5 • 6 • 7 • 8 • 9 • 10 GREAT

Actions We Should Take

_____
_____
_____
_____
_____
_____
_____
_____
_____
_____

Questions to Consider

A. Are we positive our strategy is meeting the needs of the market(s) we serve?

☐ YES • ☐ NO

B. Are we open to better ways of doing things?

☐ YES • ☐ NO

C. Can we make adjustments in our strategy quickly?

☐ YES • ☐ NO

D. Do we allow competitive forces to distract us from what we consider a solid strategy?

☐ YES • ☐ NO

E. Is meeting the needs of our patients the foundation of our strategy?

☐ YES • ☐ NO

F. Do we take calculated risks?

☐ YES • ☐ NO

Actions We Should Take

_____

_____

_____

_____

_____

_____

_____

_____

Does our internal structure support our purpose, culture, and strategy?

We clearly know our purpose, define our culture, and are confident in our strategy, and it is essential that our internal structure supports our growth as a business.

Having a professionally trained, competent, patient-focused staff using effective and efficient processes will create success beyond our highest expectations.

In my opinion, our current status is

POOR   1 • 2 • 3 • 4 • 5 • 6 • 7 • 8 • 9 • 10   GREAT

Actions We Should Take

_____

_____

_____

_____

_____

_____

_____

_____

_____

_____

_____

_____

Questions to Consider

A. Do we have a written job description for every position in the office?

☐ YES • ☐ NO

B. Do we have a performance agreement with every employee?

☐ YES • ☐ NO

C. Does every employee have an understanding of his/her job responsibilities?

☐ YES • ☐ NO

D. Are the skills of our employees matched with their position?

☐ YES • ☐ NO

E. Do we provide skills development?

☐ YES • ☐ NO

F. Do we provide self-improvement development?

☐ YES • ☐ NO

G. Are our processes patient-friendly?

☐ YES • ☐ NO

H. Is it easy to do business with us?

☐ YES • ☐ NO

Actions We Should Take

_____

_____

_____

_____

Do we deliver superior patient service?

The most significant factor that determines the success of our office is the level of patient service we provide. Superior patient service begins with the doctor and extends to the entire team.

Many dental offices say they deliver superior patient service. The important voice is the patient's—what do our patients say about our services? Research shows that 68% of the patients who quit doing business with a particular dental office do so because of the indifference shown to them by a team member of that office. In other words, they believe the dental office doesn't care about them and they go in search of a dental office that will appreciate them.

Research also shows that it takes five times more effort to obtain a new patient than to retain one. The good news is that with the level of poor patient service in the marketplace, there is a huge window of opportunity to retain and obtain patients when you make them your number one priority.

In my opinion, our current status is
POOR   1 • 2 • 3 • 4 • 5 • 6 • 7 • 8 • 9 • 10   GREAT

Actions We Should Take

_____
_____
_____
_____
_____

Questions to Consider

A. Is our patient our top priority?

☐ YES • ☐ NO

B. By our deeds and actions, do we demonstrate that our patient is "king"?

☐ YES • ☐ NO

C. Does everyone in the dental office realize they are in patient service?

☐ YES • ☐ NO

D. Do we spend more effort obtaining new patients than retaining existing patients?

☐ YES • ☐ NO

E. Are our policies, procedures, and processes "patient-friendly"?

☐ YES • ☐ NO

F. Are our team members empowered to resolve patient dissatisfaction?

☐ YES • ☐ NO

Actions We Should Take

_____

_____

_____

_____

_____

_____

What are the profiles of our best patients?

The standard rule of thumb, as they say, is that 20% of our patients provide 80% of our revenues. You can break this rule. First, determine what characteristics you want in your best patients. Second, match those characteristics with the patients you have. Odds are, most of those will be in the 20% category. Third, work hard to retain those patients while still putting your efforts into obtaining more like them.

In my opinion, our current status is
POOR   1 • 2 • 3 • 4 • 5 • 6 • 7 • 8 • 9 • 10   GREAT

Characteristics of Our Best Patients

_____
_____
_____
_____
_____
_____
_____
_____
_____
_____
_____
_____

Questions to Consider

A. Are we aware of who our best patients are?

☐ YES • ☐ NO

B. Have we identified the characteristics of the patients we want to retain and obtain?

☐ YES • ☐ NO

C. Does 80% of our business come from 20% of our patients?

☐ YES • ☐ NO

Characteristics of Our Best Patients

_____

_____

_____

_____

_____

_____

_____

_____

_____

_____

_____

_____

Do we communicate effectively with our patients?

The three C's of communication are: clear, concise, and consistent. The key is to evaluate our services from the end user's perspective. What will motivate the patient to use our services over another dental office? One of the best sources of valid information is to ask them—ask them in the office, mail them a survey, email them an online survey, or use other research procedures. Once we know what they need or want we can craft our message to communicate how to meet their needs. To communicate effectively with our patients we need a carefully crafted message that is clear, concise, and consistent. Then, we match our message to the media that is targeted to the profile of our best patients.

In my opinion, our current status is
POOR   1 • 2 • 3 • 4 • 5 • 6 • 7 • 8 • 9 • 10   GREAT

Actions We Should Take

_____
_____
_____
_____
_____
_____
_____

Questions to Consider

A. Do we have a clear, concise, and consistent message to convey to patients?

☐ YES • ☐ NO

B. Do we communicate the benefits of our services from the patient's perspective?

☐ YES • ☐ NO

C. Does our entire team know what message to communicate?

☐ YES • ☐ NO

D. Have we asked our patients, "How can we better serve you?"

☐ YES • ☐ NO

E. Does our message provide a solution?

☐ YES • ☐ NO

F. Does our message evoke a response?

☐ YES • ☐ NO

Actions We Should Take

_____

_____

_____

_____

_____

_____

_____

_____

Are we maximizing the use of available technology for business solutions?

For many of us, the "technology evolution" is both exciting and confusing. Technology is only valuable when we can use it for business solutions. Technology now gives us the tools to find solutions to our challenges and opens a world of opportunities. If we are going to survive in business today and tomorrow, we must have people with highly technical skills on our staff, yet a large number of dentists spend the least amount on technology.

In my opinion, our current status is
POOR   1 • 2 • 3 • 4 • 5 • 6 • 7 • 8 • 9 • 10   GREAT

New Ways We Can Use Technology

_____
_____
_____
_____
_____
_____
_____
_____
_____
_____

Questions to Consider

A. Is all of our staff technologically competent?
   ☐ YES • ☐ NO

B. Is someone keeping a watchful eye on changing technology so that we are not derailed off the fast track?
   ☐ YES • ☐ NO

C. Are we using technology for business solutions?
   ☐ YES • ☐ NO

New Ways We Can Use Technology

_____
_____
_____
_____
_____
_____
_____
_____
_____
_____
_____
_____

"What if...?"

"What if...?" questions are designed to help prepare us for effectively handling a possible challenge or maximizing an opportunity well in advance of the actual occurrence. A "What if...?" question challenges us to draw on all of our experiences and get our creative juices flowing. By anticipating and preparing for a situation, we can more positively affect an outcome.

In my opinion, our current status is

POOR   1 • 2 • 3 • 4 • 5 • 6 • 7 • 8 • 9 • 10   GREAT

Ask Yourself, "What if ... ?"

_____

_____

_____

_____

_____

_____

Ask Yourself, "What if ... ?"

_____

_____

_____

_____

_____

_____

Questions to Consider

A. Do we frequently ask "What if...?" questions?
   ☐ YES • ☐ NO

B. Are we aware of factors that could have a significant positive or negative impact on our office?
   ☐ YES • ☐ NO

C. Are we prepared for the possibility of a significant impact on our office?
   ☐ YES • ☐ NO

Ask Yourself, "What if ... ?"

_____
_____
_____
_____
_____
_____

Ask Yourself, "What if ... ?"

_____
_____
_____
_____
_____
_____

Are we retaining existing patients and obtaining new ones?

The best measurement of the success of our office is a quantitative report each month tracking the number of current active patients and new patients obtained during the month. The implication here is not that patients are just numbers but what those numbers represent. An increase in both categories most likely indicates we are meeting our patients' needs. A decrease in both categories most likely indicates that we are not meeting their needs. While you can't take these numbers as proof positive, you will detect trends. With computer technology, even in a large dental office, we should be able to generate some form of tracking report.

In my opinion, our current status is
POOR   1 • 2 • 3 • 4 • 5 • 6 • 7 • 8 • 9 • 10   GREAT

I think we can retain more patients if we

_____

_____

_____

_____

_____

_____

_____

_____

Questions to Consider

A. Do we measure the number of patients we retain and obtain every month?

☐ YES • ☐ NO

B. If a patient leaves our office, do we determine the reason why?

☐ YES • ☐ NO

C. Do we have a follow-up procedure to if we lose a patient?

☐ YES • ☐ NO

D. Do we have a follow-up procedure to welcome newly obtained patients?

☐ YES • ☐ NO

I think we can obtain more patients if we

_____
_____
_____
_____
_____
_____
_____
_____
_____

Thoughts and Ideas

Conclusion

In summary, I have talked about the importance of leadership and the way that effective leaders communicate and get everyone on board. I have suggested that 80% of the office is run by the employees and that great employees create a great work environment. Without an effective team, we would not be able to function, and every single doctor needs to understand that fact.

- Coach Ike Rahimi, DMD

About the Author

Hi! My name is Ike Rahimi, and I obtained my degree in Doctor of Medicine in Dentistry from the University of Pennsylvania. Soon after graduation, I bought a small practice and transformed it into a successful, thriving, and award-winning dental office.

By mastering the ability to wear different hats (CEO, CFO, Office Manager, HR Manager, and Sales & Marketing Manager) and continuing to work as a practicing clinician who knows the ins and outs of a good dental business model, I obtained first-hand knowledge in creating an award winning dental office. Consequently, through overcoming difficult challenges, I have created a proven management system.

Thoughts and Ideas

Thoughts and Ideas